FROM FLAB TO ABS

DR. LIMITLESS J.A. WILLIAMS

FROM FLAB TO ABS

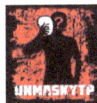

UNMASKYTP

211 POUNDS AND 31% BODY FAT

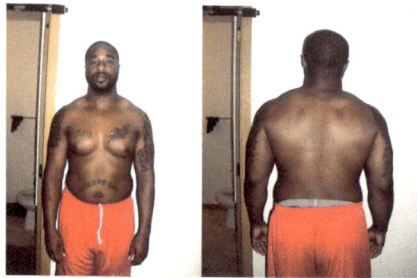

SEPTEMBER 13, 2025
OVERALL MEN'S CLASSIC PHYSIQUE

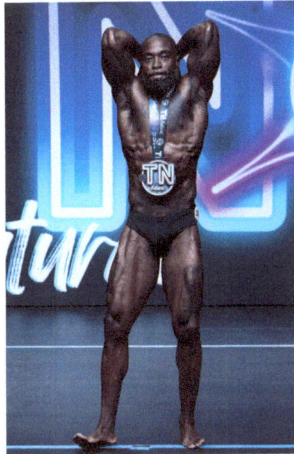

Dedication

To all who aspire to build a limitless body by strengthening the mind, awakening the spirit, and mastering the emotions.
This journey is for those who choose discipline over comfort, growth over fear, and purpose over excuses.

CONTENTS

INTRODUCTION

M ost people want to have their cake and eat it to. To me, this is a no brainer because I do want cake and want to eat it to. The conundrum is I have a strong desire for abs and a healthy vessel. I want hard abs that exhibit ripples when I wear tight-fitted shirts. I want people to witness my hard work in the gym and self-discipline in the kitchen. That is a lie, there is a slight bit of vanity that want other people to admire my cuts and to view me as some demigod. I think that is a bit much, but I am sure you understand my thought process. It is hard to have the hard physique and abs when you lust after food constantly throughout the day. My lust led me to eat donuts, honey buns, cakes, and anything sweet that pique my interest. I had a love affair with sugar; I would salivate when I wife removed cakes or cupcakes from our oven. I am still a glutton for carbohydrates (carbs) and breads which can produce flab and hide abs.

Over the years, I fell in love with Club crackers, brownies, and Nothing Bundt cakes. I lived for food, and I still love food. I have a radical acceptance of that pleasant truth. Food is a part of life, and we should not fear food, even the sugary, processed, and bad carbs. However, food should not control our lives or serve as our motivator to live. Food started to control me, and there were many nights that I wondered off, dreaming about want I would eat the next day. I envisioned purchasing a Chick-fil-a sandwich and spreading honey mustard sauce on my bun. I would wake up, with a slight smile, just to imagine how I would devour it and shoot the wrapper in the trash can like winning the NBA finals. It was an absolute love fest. I thought about how I would wash down the taste of my sandwich and waffle fries with a chilled Dr. Pepper. My parents warned me constantly, "Limitless, you reap what you sow."

I sowed a lot of surgery and fatty seeds that stuck to the front and side handles of my abdomen. I had bloated belly and over-stretched waist. I was fluffy and round, a true "dad bod" that equated to flab. Secretly, I desired the sleek abs and so-called sexy looks, but once again, I had an adulterous love affair with food, so-called good and so-called bad. A duality existed that produced this internal conflict between my spirit and my flesh. This conflict became the nexus to my personal paradigm shift, propelling my spirit to wage war with my external shell and inciting a new pattern of actions. This transformed me to pursue the best version of me, introducing me to my mantra: Be better than your best. Some researchers have purported that 35.7% of the American population is obese or morbidly obese, indicating that a large portion of America's citizens have succumb to excuses (e.g., not having the time to work out, cannot diet or afford eating healthy food, or afford a trainer, to name a few).

This book will dispel your excuses and provide us with proven and simplistic plans to enable us to see our abs and to enhance our toned up bodies. These plans will work for the average Joe or Jane; the more you believe and commit to my plan, the more your abs will pop or your stomachs will tone up. My body is proned to developing abs, but I do not believe everyone is born to have abs. Yet, I do believe everyone could improve their physique and slim up, but more importantly, I know everyone could be healthier by making smarter decisions in the kitchen and by training and unconditionally loving their bodies. I know you are wondering what gives me credibility to speak on this manner? Who am I? How do I know my so-called simplistic plan will work for any reader? I am an average Joe, with no background in physical fitness training and no specialized knowledge that gives me some special advantage on any of you. My journey started on July 31, 2014 after I was diagnosed with hypertension, known in my family as "high blood pressure" (HBP). I was prescribed medicine by my physician, and this diagnosis led me to search for some healthier alternatives without medication. I found my healthy path and grew passionate about the fitness and food process, and 10-months later, I dropped 8 inches in my waist, 42 pounds, and 10% body fat.

Before moving forward and reading the steps that transformed my mind, body, and spirit; I encourage all of you to revisit my before and after pictures. Those pictures represent us, and what we can do when we make the conscious decision to do more and to be better. My steps are very doable, and we are very capable of transitioning from flab to abs, even if that means losing a pound or five pounds. This book should inspire progress because progress leads us to our individual best versions of ourselves. Competition is with our inner spirits and with no other being in the physical realm.

MAKE A COMMITMENT TO PHYSICAL FITNESS

All journeys must begin somewhere, and it requires a force that drives you beyond the vanity or looking great aspect of working out. An impetus this robust will push you beyond the proverbial start, and two-week stop, and poor diets that accompany the majority of the average Joe's and Jane's in typical gyms. People eat food for two reasons: benefits and pleasures. The problem is that average Joe and Jane eat for mere pleasure and very rarely for any benefits. Before I delve deeper into my journey and reasoning for committing to physical fitness and to positive living, I need to discuss the significant difference between a benefit and a pleasure in the context of eating.

A **pleasure** (an unhealthy food for the purposes of this book) is something that feeds your inner animal or fleshly desire. Sometimes pleasures can be uncontrollable, creating irresistible urges that drive you to engage in harmful behaviors. Pleasures are normally selfish pursuits, and they are not considered a significant need, even though many people will argue to the contrary because the pleasure supersedes normalcy or reality. I have sought many sinful pleasures; pleasures that led me to an abnormal belly and impulses to wake up at night and scarf down six brownies covered with vanilla ice cream or four bowls of Cinnamon Toast Crunch mixed with Frosted Flakes. As you can see, I pursued a lot of pleasures that placated my appetite rather than eating food to accommodate a healthy lifestyle or fit body.

Some of you might be asking what is wrong with eating brownies or taking on four bowls of cereal...life is short, and we must enjoy ourselves. I cannot say that I disagree. On the contrary, I agree with this notion. Pleasures are not ideal when you are fighting an abnormal size, obesity, or delving in those high caloric pleasures daily, especially if you have a sedentary lifestyle—live for the TV, and the TV waits patiently for your beaming eyes. I have learned that you can enjoy pleasures while eliminating fat and building muscle by taking an advantage of benefits.

A **benefit** (a healthy food for purposes of this book) serves as a necessary boon to healthy living and an amazing physique that turns heads on the regular—you should be smiling and imaging a life with both—it is very possible, and you will have it. Benefits are essential to a life of wellbeing. Benefits provide the significant vitamins and nutrients required to fight common colds, cancer cells, and other health-related issues. Benefits also provide individuals with the robust foundation required to pack on muscle and cut exorbitant amounts of body fat in short spans of time. I am speaking from experience and lessons I implemented that cut my weight by 40 pounds and 8% body fat in 7 months. I hope I gained your attention and rejuvenated your psyche to benefits and my philosophy to health and abs.

Benefits create a healthy balance between our proverbial wants and needs. What are our wants and needs? I know you are thinking of it, and you are correct; the wants are our pleasures and the needs are our benefits. My description of wants and needs provide you with a parochial perspective of our pursuit of pleasures and benefits. A tasty Krispy Kreme donut provides your body with about 180 calories with a high dose a sugar intake, no significant protein gains, and exorbitant grams of fat; this is an absolute pleasure that and no positive gains to your health and body, unless you are seeking a smile and a salivating taste. A simplistic formula that I have adopted from friends who are dietitians is to view food with double-digit grams in protein, single-digit grams in sugars and fats as benefits, and view foods as pleasures when single-digit grams represent proteins and double-digit grams represent sugars and fats. Revisiting the Krispy Kreme donut, a pack of tuna gives the body about 20 grams of protein, 0 grams of sugar and 1.5 grams of fat; it only equates for about 70 calories—this is definitely a benefit to our bodies.

CHAPTER

3

WHAT IS YOUR MOTIVATION?

This question must be answered honestly before you can make any substantial and life altering progress. Without a strong enough purpose, your pursuit and journey to health and abs will fail. Your reason might be very logical in your mind, such as getting ready for the summer, fitting in some wedding dress, or wearing some jeans from high school. Those are great sub goals, but you will ultimately fail and regress if that serves as the reasoning or real motivator behind your pursuit. You might be wondering what is my reasoning because the title of the book states how to get abs and eat like a fat boy, but both of those were my sub goals while the true motivation was poor health, rather than a fit physique and rock hard abs. I was diagnosed with high blood pressure, and I accepted this fate—my mom and two brothers were diagnosed, so I conceded to the idea of this being hereditary. I surmised that the medical doctors and researchers must be correct in this manner.

I went along with their medical regiment, and I proceeded to consume chlorothiazide within the parameters of their prescribed dosage, accepting my fate as a blood pressure (BP) patient for life at the age of 34. You should be able to feel the melancholy resonated in my writing; it was a sad and depressing diagnosis to accept. Yet, I found peace with the corollary of fighting to reduce my high blood pressure readings. As I commenced to take my medicine, I noticed that my equilibrium was off...fighting random dizzy spells, and I had constant blurred vision and became tired easily. The cumbersome side effects were creating an upheaval in my life and sapping me of my positive energy and spirit. Something had to change—medicine would no longer be the solution for my BP, but I had no alternative solution.

This conundrum was the impetus to my lifestyle change, and it drove me to explore potential solutions and awakening this trained researcher within me by vetting over scientific manuscripts, studying opinionated responses or thoughts, and testing all of these theories that made sense to me. I am a scholar and researcher by profession, but we are all born to be innate researchers and thinkers, exploring an insatiable thirst for answers as infants and toddlers once exiting our mothers' wombs. When challenges or daily obstacles impede our progression in any form, it is an opportunity for growth and resolutions that can augment our lifestyles. It starts with our minds—viewing the obstacle as a negative or a positive. Being sick and diagnosed with high hypertension was viewed as a positive, and yes, I called BP a sickness; we tend to view anything outside the norm as abnormal, so hypertension is considered the opposite of healthy.

I had an irresistible desire to be healthy, and I truly believed that God would allow me to be healthy. I no longer bought into the idea of surviving with manufactured pills that were produced in pharmaceutical plants to precise measurements. It was driven by a question that would never leave my mind: how did people survive and thrive in ancient times before pharmaceutical plants and quality assurance specialists? Prompting me to research ancient African proverbs, Moorish societies, Spain's medicine (Renaissance Period), and primitive medical measures during the maturation of America. All of this information led me to the Hippocratic oath, and it helped me devise this following summation and separation from seeking medicine to sustain and improve our lives:

"Respect the sages who prepare you to serve others, serve patients with respect and perform service with due diligence. Do not put patient in harm or injustice, treating them equality. Respect the rights of patients by keeping them informed and being ethical at all times. Do not intimidate patients, and try to prevent as well as cure all diseases. Provide confidentiality to all patients, and impart your medical knowledge and advice to all of your patients and individuals".

I want to draw your attention to the lines to "prevent as well as cure all diseases" and to "impart your medical knowledge and advice to all of your patients and individuals". These lines infused me to find a solution to hypertension because my prescribed medicine was not the panacea and failed to prevent or cure my sickness—medicine actually made me feel physically worse. My insatiable desire to learn medical knowledge and possible resolutions led me to the following three essential motivating elements for my lifestyle transformation:

1. We must believe that we were crafted for greatness.
2. We must be willing to commit to a healthy lifestyle—not any temporary change.

3. We must be able to visualize a rock hard and tone body that our eyes never imagined or have seen.

These vital elements will lead us to a healthy body that will last a lifetime. Both were acquired while I still ate like a fat boy. The unspoken question in many of our minds and ultimately hearts is, "how did I accomplish this amazingly and seemingly impossible feat"? First of all, I did not accomplish this exuberating endeavor by thinking like that, on the contrary, I believed beyond belief; and I refused to accept defeat or any other outcome—toned abs and medicine free were the only two outcomes—no compromising.

BELIEVE IN A FORCE THAT IS GREATER THAN US

W e must believe that we were crafted for greatness and the image of perfection; that image must be contrived in our minds and must penetrate the depths of our hearts—and rest in our hearts throughout the entire transformation. This is a process, and the process always begins in our minds, travels to our hearts, and then it develops into an irresistible passion that drives us beyond our mere human efforts and powers. The previous declaration is the reason why we must rely on a force much greater than us because we will stop and complain, finding a myriad of reasons to stymie the process and to regress further from toned abs and a healthy state of well-being. I am speaking from experience, so I encourage all of you to thinking about past failures. How many excuses did you make for your shortcomings? I realized the more reasons or excuses I found, the longer I played the victim and the longer I veered off the right path. We all veer off path from time-to-time, but please do not be dismayed; we must dig deeper and use a greater force to pull us to something greater.

We can conceive that concept by examining the theory behind Newton's laws. Newton's laws explained gravity as a force that attracts a body of mass to the center of the earth, or towards any other body having mass. The core of our vessels or flesh has a desire-seeking mechanism that is contrived in our hearts. This desire-seeking mechanism magnetizes things toward us to placate our center, and our center attempts to appease the core or heart of our beliefs. Our beliefs dictate the corollary, and our beliefs are responsible for the design of our appearance, attitude, and actions. All positive outcomes flock to positive people; success draws to successful thinkers, and the more success one acquires, the more one expects to acquire. Some might question the authenticity of this statement because you might suggest that negative people acquire success; and I agree that they can set a goal and accomplish it. However, I do not believe it will be sustainable or positive.

For example, we can examine the following two scenarios about these individuals who loss a significant amount of weight; they both accomplished their goals, but only one of them found positive outcomes. Scenario one focuses on Roger Clemens who used drug enhancements to perform and play major league baseball at an extremely high level. Roger was blessed with amazing talents that gave him the strength to throw curves and fastballs from the pitcher mound, and he worked diligently to augment his talents and amplify his performance on the baseball field. Enabling him to acquire massive successes and exorbitant wealth throughout the longevity of his career. However, his unethical behavior or illicit drug use (a negative) caused him to lure in negative consequences. He ruined his career and, people turned against him and questioned his character. Sadly, the Hall of Fame committee is shunning him for his past behaviors and mistakes.

Scenario two is about Tony Dungy, a man who employs his belief in God as the impetus for his decision-making as a coach and in his every day life. He attempted to emulate the life of Jesus, so he made a point of treating his players with the upmost respect and drafting and signing players of high character, to create a positive and loving environment. He never compromised on his values, even when he was fired as a successful head coach of the Tampa Bay Buccaneers. He held his head high and continued to practice what he preached when he became the official head coach of the Indianapolis Colts. Acquiring a multitude of successes, most noticeably, becoming the first black head football coach to win a Super Bowl and posting many regular season best records. Most importantly, he has distinguished himself as an individual with high character, attaining success and positive outcomes (e.g., high integrity and moral character).

These scenarios demonstrate the significance of believing in something greater than self. In my opinion, Roger Clemens' actions derived from the belief in self, and Tony Dungy's attitude and actions originated from his belief in a higher power. What does this have to do with my plight to a healthy lifestyle and toned abs? My attitude towards eating and working out improved, and my pursuit to significant weight loss and abs became possible when I made my belief in God the focal point. Prior to this approach, I worked out solely for vanity reasons or short-term goals, which in-turn, never made working out and conscious eating (e.g., reading labels and being aware of sodium and caloric intake) a lifestyle. I would workout for hours and witness minimal results because it was about me, not about a sacrifice or glory to God. Yet, my paradigm shifted when I was diagnosed with hypertension and medicine failed to rectify my dire situation.

I stated dire because I had high blood pressure readings of 180/110; and the medicine lowered my blood pressure but created dizzy spells and blurred vision, making me feel worse and incapable of performing specific fitness or reading related tasks at times. When I entered my new workout facility in Knoxville, TN on September 15, 2014, I entered with a new paradigm to get healthy and to decrease my body fat to honor and to glorify God. Believing that I was made in God's perfect image and made for greatness, I began to believe that I could procure excellence in my overall wellness—mind, body, and spirit. My actions started to mirror a positive attitude towards excellence. I believed I was destined for ripped abs, and a life free of legalized prescription drugs. This belief was anchored in my willingness to emulate a life exemplary of Christ's principles.

PRINCIPLES GOVERNING MY EATING AND WORKOUTS

"Do you not know that your bodies are temples of the Holy Spirit, who is in you, whom you have received from God? You are not your own;" 1 Corinthians 6:19

My paradigm shifted from an egocentric focus to an honor God focus. I no longer considered glorifying myself with selfish wants of shaping my body like guys from fitness magazines; I wanted to be healthy and present an image that God designed specifically for me—a body free of medicine and toned to the likeness of God. I truly believed it was possible if I removed my selfish desires from the equation and focused on listening to the quiet inner voice that I coined as God. Initially, it is hard to create and maintain this high level of focus until I continued to pray and make God the nucleus or reasoning behind every meal and every workout. The above scripture came alive in me, and it inspired me adopt this lifestyle philosophy; the belief in something greater than self is essential to the understanding of self and to the hidden motivation needed to aggrandize self. When I embraced this new outlook on eating and working out, I realized that I did not have all the answers; and that the truth to health and to abs will come from multiple sources—people, books, documentaries, web searches, my inner voice, and unfamiliar workouts and foods outside my proverbial norm.

I had to debunk all my previous myths, be open-minded, and believe the so-called impossible, knowing that impossible translates to a code word I contrived called "Imakeepossible" (I make everything possible). Making things possible can only happen with an open-mind, realizing that we do not know everything, and we should never be the smartest individual in every room; we must embrace the ideal that something new can be learned in every encounter—always seek new knowledge; this life lesson is a must as we evolve, personally and professionally. My journey commenced with my daily food intake. I had to evaluate what I was eating and why I was eating certain foods. My colleagues, Kiwon and Lee educated me about my caloric intake, good carbs and fats, bad carbs and fats, water intake, healthy snacks, how often to eat, and the importance of protein. I randomly would solicit advice from fitness trainers and fitness models sauntering throughout my workout locale.

Information is free and random, and information enabled me to reach my individual excellence. I was conversing with my older brother about my lifestyle change, and he casually informed me about a documentary *Forks Over Knives*. This documentary spoke about America's massive consumption of meats, sugars, and diary products, illustrating an exorbitant consumption of meats and processed foods since the 1900's. Prompting me to alter my diet and take up a vegan diet for about two months, only deviating from that diet once a week for lean protein: packed tuna and veggie chips. Below is an example of my vegan diet, which I kept below 1500-1700 calories:

My First Daily Diet / Routine

Time	Meal / Activity
6:00 AM	Half bottle of water (500 ml) and a five-minute meditation
7:00 AM	One piece of fruit (cutie/orange, apple, or banana) and finish the remaining 500 ml of water
9:30 AM	After returning from the gym: salad with beans (protein), fruit, other vegetables, and balsamic vinaigrette; drink another bottle of water (500 ml)
11:00 AM	Snack on almonds (read label and limit to 150 calories); stay within a daily range of 1500–1700 calories; drink another bottle of water (500 ml)
1:30 PM	Bag of vegetables (broccoli, carrots, celery, tomatoes); optional small amount of dressing—read the label and stay within calorie range; drink another bottle of water (500 ml or 17 oz)
4:00 PM	Hummus and carrots (no more than 150 calories); remain within the 1500–1700 calorie limit; drink another bottle of water (500 ml or 17 oz)
7:00 PM	Hearty vegetable soup and vegetables of choice; drink a bottle of water (500 ml or 17 oz)
9:00 PM	Green tea and water before bed; if hungry, eat one boiled egg and remove the yolk before sleeping

I must mention that we might need to adjust our caloric-intakes to match our body types. For example, a small petite female may need to limit her calories to 1200 per day, while a larger male may need to limit his calories to 1800 per day. On my plan, we should never consume more than 1500-1700 calories while we are attempting to lose weight on my plan, even during our cheat day or cheat meal...no exceptions to this rule. Every day we should be consuming six bottles of water (120ml) or more and do not incorporate juice until recommended. Periodically, we have moments of hunger for about a week and a half until our bodies begin to adjust to this new way of living. Our bodies are conditioned to eat more than it needs to survive. This intense diet will reteach our bodies to accept the appropriate portion size and shrink our stomachs to a capacity that can hold small portions of food at any given time. Note...we should be working out while integrating this diet to see our maximum results, and we should stick to my workout plan. We will discuss my workout plan throughout the remainder of this book.

This diet might be a little intense, boring, and hard for most picky eaters or stubborn-minded individuals. However, my results demonstrate a positive output, and I highly recommend that we attempt a vegan diet for a month with one cheat day. During your cheat day, you can consume what you desire, even sweets; but you must not take your calories over the 1500-1700 calories threshold. This threshold must not be exceeded even if we have to cut some meals throughout the day to remain under this caloric number...**DO NOT EXCEED 1500-1700 calories.** It is pertinent to partake in this diet because it will make the vegetarian and my typical eating style more rewarding and enjoyable; it will help your mind fall in love with this healthy eating process.

My vegan diet accompanies my beginner workout regiment, and they are both used to ease me into the process while seeing significant gains early in this process.

This method bolstered the momentum I needed to stay focused and to start falling in love with this unusual workout and eating affair. Initial workouts might be a little daunting for you, and you might even be a little lethargic in the gym—stick with it and do not give up. All of my workouts consist of this simple rule of thumb: **40-45 minutes of weight training and 20-25 minutes of cardio training**. Now, my workouts might last as long as two hours if I play some games of basketball; as you get stronger and more fit, you should judge your body and decide training intervals for yourself. I adopted this rule of thumb from some of the best professional football and basketball players. However, I will explain the basic science behind it. Our bodily tissues use this substance called glycogen (a short-term storage form of carbohydrates) during the first 40-45 minutes of our workouts—giving us the energy, strength, and the overall push needed to throw around weights in the gym. After we burn through glycogen, our body decides to burn the fat off our physiques, prompting me to employ cardio to target the fat.

A trainer named Joe Dodgin informed me that people typically lose fat where they gained fat deposits first. I tend to believe and support his notion because my fat melted away from the front and side of my beer belly first. This method sheds fats and tones those fat areas—I started to see results within the first three weeks.

Below, I will construct a typical beginner workout:

My Beginner Workout

Workouts should be used to give you an idea of what might work for you. The best workouts are ones contrived to fit your personal interest; they should be challenging, rewarding, and fun...yes...fun.

Warm-up for five minutes on the arc trainer or recumbent bike. Choose a machine of your liking to make sure that you warm-up appropriately. Try to loosen up all muscles during this session. Now that you are ready to train, I will provide you with a beginner workout to get you progression towards health, cut abs, and a toned body. Every workout is performed with 12-15 repetitions (reps); however, notice that some series are performed with 8-10 reps. Do not give yourself more than 20 seconds to rest after performing an exercise...stay busy and keep moving.

Note:

You should remain in the zone throughout the duration of your workout. For example, your triceps should be feeling the burn for the entire extension or exercise.

Find your appropriate weight or adjust weight to meet the reps of your desire for every workout listed below:

BEGINNER WORKOUT PROGRAM

MONDAY – BICEPS & SHOULDERS

Note: The first set of all biceps exercises is always 20 reps.

Biceps & Shoulders Workout

Exercise	Sets	Reps	Notes
Standing Cable Bicep Curls (squeeze at peak)	1	20	Focus on contraction
	2	12–15	Increase weight each set
Concentration Curls (arm over incline bench)	1	20	Slow and controlled
	2	12–15	Increase weight
Alternating Dumbbell Shoulder Press	1	20	Standing or seated
	2	12–15	Increase weight
Front Shoulder Raises (straight arms)	1	20	Controlled motion
	2	12–15	Increase weight
Dumbbell Hammer Curls	1	20	Each arm
	2	12–15	Increase weight

Cardio (Post-Workout)
- Duration: **25 minutes**
- Choose a machine that allows intensity variation
- Increase intensity every 5 minutes → then decrease for 5 minutes
- Repeat until time is complete

TUESDAY – LEGS & BACK (BEGINNER)

Exercise	Sets	Reps	Notes
Seated Leg Press	1	25	Controlled tempo
	2	12–15	Increase weight
Standing Speed Squats	3	12–15	Explosive but controlled
Alternating Lunges	3	12–15 each leg	Maintain balance
Leg Extensions	1	20	Each leg
	2	12–15	Increase weight
Standing Dumbbell Calf Raises	1	20	Full stretch
	2	12–15	Increase weight

WEDNESDAY – CARDIO & RECOVERY

No weights today.

Choose one:

- Basketball
- Racquetball
- Tennis
- Treadmill
- Stair climber (highly recommended)
- Arc trainer
- Outdoor running

Intensity Rule (Talk Test):

You should be **too out of breath to sing**, but able to say a few words.

Use **intervals**:

- Push hard

- Recover briefly
- Repeat

Listen to your body and learn what challenges you effectively.

THURSDAY – CHEST & TRICEPS

Focus on form and the squeeze.

Exercise	Sets	Reps	Notes
Standing Straight-Bar Pushdowns	1	20	Control movement
	2	12–15	Increase weight
Single or Double Arm Kickbacks	1	20	Focus on extension
	2	12–15	Increase weight
Standing Rope Triceps Extensions	1	20	Full range
	2	12–15	Increase weight
Dips	1	15	Bodyweight
	4	12–15	Add resistance if needed

FRIDAY – CORE & CONDITIONING

(Repeat circuit 4 times)

Exercise	Reps / Time
Pull-Ups	8–10
Plank	30 seconds
V-Ups	12
Core Variations (upper, mid, lower abs)	12–15

Exercise	Reps / Time
Cardio	30 minutes

SATURDAY – OPTIONAL CARDIO

Repeat Wednesday's cardio structure:

- Sports or machine-based cardio
- Interval-based intensity
- Push until speech becomes difficult
- Rest briefly, then repeat

Listen to your body.

SUNDAY – REST & RECOVERY

Hydrate. Stretch. Recover. Prepare for the next week.

My beginner diet and workout guide was found through trial and error. I tried multiple meals and workouts until I found those that served as a boon to my mental and physical development. Both were accomplished by employing this overarching theme: "I eat to glorify God, and I worked hard to glorify God." We must embrace a mindset that enables us to equip ourselves with the discipline needed to eat appropriately and to train incessantly for excellence. Acquiring a fit muscular frame and healthy body requires our best, and our best is bolstered by a great force, not our parochial humanistic minds and perspectives. This statement should indicate to you, the reader, that my workouts and diets were contrived from an outside collaboration—a force that cannot be explained with my simple words. Depending on your beliefs, you may recognize this force as energy, religion, science, or deity. God was the force that drove me, and my fundamental belief in Jesus Christ.

My belief propelled me to excellence in the kitchen and in the gym; both are extreme challenges for most people. Obesity and juvenile diabetes are posting record numbers in America, and you can attend any city or state to witness the normalcy of Americans casually walking around unhealthy or obese. Our eyes can recognize truth in the physical; our eyes create our perception and perception becomes our reality. Most people will utilize all types of excuses to explain their morbid obesity. I have heard people on TV and in person explain an inability to work out as their reasoning, food addiction, physical disability, coping mechanism, and insufficient time. All of the excuses might be valid to your cognitive thinking capacity, but I have seen people work out on the airplane or in the snow, overcome drug addictions, climb mountains without limbs, bury family members and perform exceptionally in sporting events, and conduct 10-minute workouts, debunking all of their spoken excuses.

Those amazing individuals accomplished those wonderful feats by channeling internal powers and tapping into a power greater than self and their human efforts. It might appear that I am touting God, but I am selling you on the difficulty of adopting a healthy lifestyle without a belief in something greater than self; it makes the plight darn near impossible. My many years of bad eating and lack of gains in the gym have provided me with the insight to make the previous declarations—I fully understand the wrong way of living and the fit way of living—drug free and tight abs flexing. Our underlying principles can make us extraordinary when it comes to eating and workout and shifts our paradigms from a sedentary one to a "busy bee".

BE A BUSY BEE

B ees are annoying to humans because they are very active and noisy. Bees work incessantly to produce honey and bees wax, and they are vital to pollination. Bees unmatched work ethic drive most situations crazy as they fly around our ears and head, causing us to emote with flailing arms and irritating screams. This brings me to the notion of "busy bees" or hyper humans who never stop moving or working; these individuals annoy many humans with their incessant behavior. Yet, being a busy bee provides one with a mentality needed to stay engaged to the work out process. We learn to keep moving and view working out as something that needs to be constant, becoming an essential part of our lifestyles—on par with brushing teeth and washing our private parts. I start every day fresh, and I begin every day with a workout and renewed slate to my physical fitness.

Starting fresh gave me an opportunity to ask these questions: what can I learn new today, how can I glorify God with my workouts, food, and positive energy, and what can I do to make this transformation process a fun experience? The way I live is similar to the way I design peer-reviewed articles; I employ questions to guide my purpose in every day because there are central questions that guide thought-provoking research. Questions keep me busy and explorative, so I find myself evaluating opportunities to transform my body and thinking in multiple situations, maximizing majority of my time in a constructive manner. For example, I might be sitting on the floor watching some show on *Investigative Discovery* when I quietly ask myself what can I be doing to augment my body—maybe some crunches or maybe some push-ups. The more I ask those internal questions, the more my internal fire grows towards a transformative-healthy lifestyle. What you believe is what you tend to attract.

The law of attraction is a great lesson that I learned from reading the *Secret*. The Bible also purports that a man is what a man thinks (Proverbs 27:3), so I contrived a mindset that made healthy thinking and fitness applicable to all aspects of my life. I found a way to incorporate fitness into my relationships (i.e., family and friends) and fun activities (e.g., watching TV, playing video games, reading books, and eating food). Some of you might be thinking that this is obsessive to constantly think about working out, but you need to remember, I had the mentality of a fat boy; and I am not using fat boy as a derogatory term. I define fat boy as a mentality to live to eat, and my hedonistic existence of food superseded a commitment to health and fitness. When my paradigm was programmed to fat boy status, I tended to be lazy and rather eat a plate of brownies than veggies and working out. The pleasure of moist brownies warmed with a scoop ice cream and chocolate syrup served as a form of catharsis in my life, continuing to eat even though my stomach reached its limits.

As a fat boy, it is easy to become lethargic and to accept a sedentary lifestyle, while a busy bee repudiates laziness and embodies an active mentality and constantly moving lifestyle. It is hard to satisfy the mindset of a busy bee, and it is easy to develop an insatiable hunger to work out. This ambitious attitude can also lead to potential problems—too much of anything can be bad, especially when it becomes too much about you. This is why we must be removed from this equation; it must be focused on a force greater than self. Things must be pursued in moderation—being a busy bee is no exception to the rule. I will provide three easy tactics to make being a busy bee a natural attitude to a toned body and healthy lifestyle: Practice moderation/meditation, eat in moderation during festive events, and learn to meditate and eat great.

PRACTICE MODERATION
AND MEDITATION

M ediation and moderation should be mutually exclusive tactics. When applied together, they have the power to promote and maintain a healthy lifestyle. Healthy eating and gym commitment follows a healthy lifestyle, and a healthy lifestyle is your only guarantee to a lifetime commitment of health and well-chiseled abs. Mediation requires one to think deeply and focus ones' mind for a period of time. African Proverbs and seers suggest that mediation allows individuals to tap into higher levels of thought that invoke a spiritual awakening and enlightenment of self. An understanding of self gives individuals the power needed to push beyond self-doubt, allowing individuals to walk by faith and not by sight to some unimaginable goal.

Some people consider mediation as their quiet time, and as a time to separate from others and this physical world, traveling mentally to a place outside of their physical reality. Using mediation to provide transparency into their inner thought-process or a clear purpose to their daily direction. An abstruse direction emerges when our minds our clouded with distractions (e.g., daily tasks, others' opinions, or obstacles). For example, if someone attempts to add new furniture to a house that is cluttered with debris and remnants of clothes on the floor, he or she would find it extremely difficult to position their furniture appropriately. Our minds are seeking novel ideas and facts on a regular basis, being our house that stores new furniture and augments our presentation. With a clean and clear house, we can easily annex furniture; which is synonymous to a transparent or lucid thought-process that amplifies knowledge. Meditation serves as a cog to the wheels of innovative, critical, and rational thought.

For me to build a well-defined temple that will last the duration of my existence, I needed a lucid perspective to incorporate a healthy lifestyle. A lifestyle that features an eradication of fried foods and saturated pork, as well as limited red meats, sugars, breads, and pastas. I transitioned from a reckless and food-seeking method, to a more conscious and well-disciplined pupil of health awareness and wellness. Meditation is also the catalyst to comprehending and eating in moderation. Meditation guided me to relaxation practices and focused my thinking to healthy eating. I was transformed into a sentient being; a being that was able to connect the dots between the mass consumption of food and poor health when physical activity is non-existent or minuscule.

My culture, community, and the US at large promote this "more is bigger and better" mentality; and this mentality metastasizes a mass consumption of food and overindulgence in high caloric desserts, sugary sodas, and tantalizing chocolates. An environment of this magnitude can create a toxic mass consumption attitude, becoming pervasive for generations in families and small communities. Negative or positive, attitudes, behaviors, and values are contagious and impact their immediate milieu. It is normal to find children who struggle with obesity being accompanied by parents who fight overweight issues. My mass consumption of food and lack of self-controlled can be traced throughout my lineage. Eating big meals and high caloric options were tied to festive events, love, laughter, and a slew of ignorance to this destructive lifestyle.

Partaking in the food was a tacit agreement of love and friendship in my populous. I can confidently state this practice is normal with many families throughout the U.S. Individuals will eat and eat until their stomachs are packed tight with fried foods, cakes, sodas or alcoholic beverages, breads, cheeses, and other pastries; and we can throw in a little bit of vegetables, but those vegetables are normally saturated with sugars and salt. I mentioned a lot of great tasting foods, but I did not allude to many healthy delicacies on our unstructured menu. Our eating style was a free for all, and most eat until we feel tight (belly feels as if it will burst). It was an anomaly for individuals to reject this buffet style preference; and people will taunt you for this aberration.

Loving family members and friends will ask you a bevy of questions broaching your lack of desire for their food or food being displayed: Are you on a diet? Are you too good for my food? Why are you acting shy? Why are you going to disrespect my mother's cooking? Why are you not eating more? With the constant barrage of questions and tempting items, I will eventually cave into their peer pressure, finding myself an hour later rubbing my belly and struggling to keep my eyes open. It was nothing to consume 3,000-4,000 calories during this endeavor and following that poor decision up with inertia and a realm of laziness. Yet, I would never discourage you from enjoying time with your family and friends, but I will encourage you to eat in moderations and work out prior to engaging in that destructive endeavor.

EAT IN MODERATION
DURING FESTIVE EVENTS

———————————

T he most important and logical step is to understand yourself
and your limits. You might be thinking, what the hell do I
mean by that statement? I mean you must if you are prone to over
eat during those festive events or have the proclivity to drink;
both are poor decisions and both lead to destructive behaviors
that can impact your body in a negative way. If you are suscepti-
ble to one of these actions, you must acknowledge it prior to big
gatherings. Those gatherings can be eating out at restaurants,
family reunions, and any other functions that generate massive
amounts of food. I am weak and tend to compromise during festive events, so I employ two tricks that serve as a food buffer.

The first tactic is to have a mental and physical workout. Mental and physical workouts should always be in concert
with each other and never be viewed as mutually exclusive tasks.
It is easy for cognitive dissonance to occur when the two perspectives are compartmentalized and seen as too separate activities.
As sentient beings, we must allow every function of our body to

be synchronized with each segment to build a productive unit. Your mind cannot yearn an abundance of food and accept gluttony as godliness but works incessantly to burn body fat and to develop a fit temple. These actions create a paradox of internal war within the individual operating in this fashion. Many people function within this madness of confusion every day, and they stand in front of their mirror puzzled by no visual gains and frustrated with the scale for no quantitative gains.

Gains and visual rewards are procured through an agreement of mind, body, and soul; the body must be in unison with the spirit to contrive a healthy lifestyle. This connection and maturation of a healthy lifestyle aid us to eat in moderation during festive events. And, many of us adore festive events, knowing that about 68.8% of the United States population is considered overweight. It is imperative to enter festive events with a game plan or strategy for eating and exiting the kitchen arena. Do not take this scheme lightly. Speaking from experience, family members and friends rush to the kitchen with focus and determination to overload their plates and select the most palatable items for their liking. When I begin my journey, I would enter my relatives and friends houses with a mental list of foods to mesh with my taste buds and squeeze in my new limited space.

My catalog of delicacies consisted of a taste of chocolate cake, baked chicken, veggies, and other miscellaneous items for the taste. Sweets are my vice or kryptonite, so I listed the chocolate numero uno on my short list of must consume foods. Prompting me to research the potential calories and sugars prior to engaging in a festive bash. I also make sure my previous meals were gobbled in moderation, following the serving guidelines and listening to my stomach; I eat until my hunger is quenched. All meals are accompanied with a full glass or bottle of water to decrease my capacity for storing food, an attempt to trick my mind in thinking I am full and not in need of any more food. Playing Jedi mind tricks with my mind, to redirect my attitude about food during the tempting jubilant moments of nourishment. My distinctive list will always include veggies; veggies are healthy and provide quality nutrients that occupy restricted capacity. My mind is constantly thinking about moderation; moderation is a lifestyle and everything about being healthy and being fit is my lifestyle. We cannot run or isolate ourselves from this notion.

My mindset propels me to a proactive outlook when it comes to eating and preparing for festive occurrences; it is the only way for me to succeed in this endeavor. I also interject additional workouts to compensate for eating during festive events or cheat meal days. Most people fail during their respective diets or pursuit of healthiness because they focus on working out and burning calories; but they neglect to develop a proactive and healthy mindset towards eating adequate and healthy cuisines. This leads to ultimately ends in unsuccessful diets, frustrations, and digressions to poor habits of eating and working out. The war starts in the mind, and I contrived successful strategies before the advent of prospective parties. I rewarded myself with the taste of foods rather than the devouring of all foods on my plate. Moderation is an action principle or task, but moderation requires additional willpower at times, so I encourage all who aspire to healthy living to incorporate meditation prior to engaging in cuisines.

LEARN TO MEDITATE AND EAT GREAT

Meditation is a way to cogitate or ponder over an action prior to fully engaging in it. Full engagement requires an agreement of mind, body, and soul; we should never attempt to separate the three. View it as the trinity of self, and no one can function effectively without it. Mind, body, and soul or spirit serves as a checks and balances system. The soul is the legislative branch were principles that govern our life is created and stored, the mind is the executive branch that decides what to think or necessary decisions for our life, and the body is the judicial branch that sets a precedents over situations that might supersede set rules...for instance when to eat bad foods or healthy foods. Meditation is my place of Zen, and it allows me to tap into all three levels.

I would encourage everyone to find a place of solitude to meditate, a place were there are minimal distractions. I tap into my place of peace in the mornings before anyone in the house awakens and on my drive to the gym and my drive to work. These experiences happen early in the AM, and I continue to meditate off and on throughout the day. It is critical to have an elevated sense of awareness throughout the day, not just at a specific time. This heightened sense of awareness enables your mental purpose to mesh appropriately with your physical needs. We need to think pleasant and healthy thoughts about ourselves, in order to magnetize those elements in the physical realm. For example, I purposely eat in moderation, minimize sugar intake, lift weights, and engage in cardiovascular exercises to stay lean and mean.

Notice the particular steps in the process, I conceptualized myself as a fit being, which prompted me to eat in a healthy fashion and to train in an incessant manner that was conducive for a well-toned mass; this is the benefits of meditation and moderation. Ameliorating any previous bad habits, from my mental status to my physical approach to training. Efficient and effective meditation and eating are exemplary actions of holiness; it is the true elevation to living a life that pleases God. This paradigm is a perspective that aligns with Christ and spiritual tenets from most religious texts. Meditation is an escape from our identified normal. Yet, meditation allows one to tap into spiritual realms that extend far beyond our physical realm, enabling us to tap into intangible elements. We must escape the corporeal to enlighten ourselves to the unimaginable.

For example, my sculpting commenced with about 16-18% body fat, so there was no abs and minimal striations on my body, making it impossible to formulate a fit body within my physical realm. I had to isolate my thinking to capture positive thoughts about an amazing body that did not exist, and I forced myself to contrive a vision so real that it awakened my mind to positive ethos in a spiritual domain unknown to my physical self. Meditation invoked spiritual omens that guided me prior to eating, aiding me to foods that benefited my sculpting process. Below is my modality of morning and eating meditation:

Morning & Eating Meditation Practice

There is no required time limit for this practice. Meditation may last anywhere from one minute to several hours, depending on your availability and intention.

Step	Practice	Description
1. Choose Your Space	Find a calm, quiet environment	Select a location free from distractions. Early morning is ideal, as it helps set the tone for the entire day.
2. Posture & Positioning	Sit comfortably with intention	Sit upright in a chair or on the floor. Extend your arms outward with palms open and facing upward toward the sky.
3. Controlled Breathing	Begin with deep, intentional breaths	Inhale slowly through your nose and exhale through your mouth. Complete three deep breaths to ground yourself.
4. Mental Clearing	Release stress and negativity	Clear your mind of worries, distractions, and negative thoughts. Remain in this space for a set time (approximately three minutes or longer).
5. Intentional Visualization	Fill your mind with positive imagery	Visualize the life, outcomes, and energy you desire. Focus on what you want to create and become.

Reflection Note

This practice can be done during your morning routine or before meals to enhance awareness, gratitude, and intentional living. Consistency matters more than duration.

I apply this principle prior to eating, envisioning the protein, calories, sugars, and etc. as a boon to my odyssey to peak fitness. The images are so compelling that I feel as if the ingredients are augmenting my body with every bite; I eat to live, but I saw food as the most essential component to my new physical fitness blue print. I learned to enjoy food and no longer perceive food as something negative, even foods that were high in sugar and sodium. No food is bad when you incorporate moderation and meditation. Mental power is the key to overcoming poor habits of scarfing down large portions of food and yielding to the temptations of so-called bad cuisines (i.e., donuts, cupcakes, soda, and etc.).

BLUEPRINT WOES

There is no infallible system, and my blueprint is not the panacea to never eating poorly again, especially if you have an affinity to devour delicious delicacies. My physical fitness apparatus was structured to serve as the impetus to my fine-tuned abs and commitment to bask at times, in great food and lose weight. Blueprints are plans that can provide solutions to problematic areas or preventive measures to potential issues. In order to succeed at enhancing your body and regulating your eating regiment, one must have a contingency plan. Effective businesses operate with a similar modality; businesses set up proactive plans to combat schemes that might fail.

Our bodies should be treated as those wealthy entities, but for some reason, we tend to isolate our health or human aspect of self from our jobs, family, money, and things. We inadvertently make those other elements in our lives more important than self, creating a devaluation of our bodies. This mentality will always lead to blueprint woes because the blueprint will never hold value if one fails to value self. Once again, an understanding of self is the cardinal rule of any life altering actions; you must change mind and spirit before you can sculpt your body and lose weight. When I deviate from my well-constructed blueprint, I always tap into my thinking and redirecting my believing to follow my path back to excellent health.

Over plan to combat your blueprint woes

Every plan needs a back a plan, and maybe, plans to back up those plans. What am I saying? I am saying that we should over-plan, and this is a cardinal tenet for all schemes in life. If I eat poorly or consume too many calories, I have trained myself to enhance my workouts; more specifically, revving up my cardio to burn additional calories for that particular day. I also decrease my caloric in-take in other meals throughout the day when I know that I will eat 15 cookies or an Oreo Molten cake from Chili's restaurant. Another plan is to work out on a day off to compensate for the surplus of calories that might have been added to my diet. My extensive or over-the-top tactic is to fast and pray for a day or two to refocus my mind, body, and spirit; I believe that this strategy rebalances my mind, body, and spirit, enabling me to remember that food is a source of survival and not mere pleasure.

A bevy of plans create peace and confidence in making healthy living a lifestyle rather than an event to for some given situation. It is easy for me to over plan because my plan is unique for my personality and training and food interest. Your goal is to read this text and employ what works and disregard information that will not work for you. We make mistakes in life when we attempt to use schemes that do not make use comfortable or happy during over transformation process; it is your goal to disengage from this way of conceptualizing working out. Working out has its onset of contingency plans. I plan workouts for days that I cannot make it to the gym or fail to venture to the gym. When it becomes a lifestyle, you find a way to work out and a way to avoid any excuses that can discourage that endeavor.

I have rudimentary workout equipment that suffices for my workout needs. I use a set of dumbbells, bands, and pull-up bar to maintain my physique; I also implement pushups, planks, and core exercises. During this daunting journey, your mind must always be focused on training the body and stretching the body, inside and outside the gym. The following are some of my recommended in-home exercises:

Bodyweight (Calisthenics) Workout – No Weights Required

Exercise	Sets	Reps / Time	Guidelines & Modifications
Push-Ups	10 sets	50 reps per set	Rest 1 minute between sets. *Beginner option:* 150–250 total reps with 30 seconds rest between sets.
Pull-Ups	4–5 sets	12–15 reps per set	Rest 1 minute between sets. *Beginner option:* 5 reps per set using assistance if needed.
Planks	4 sets	45–60 seconds	Beginners may hold for 30 seconds. Focus on core engagement and posture.

Exercise	Sets	Reps / Time	Guidelines & Modifications
Core Circuit	4 rounds	15 reps each	Perform with slow, controlled movement for full contraction: · Six-inch leg raises (15) · Mid-range leg raises (15) · Crunches (15) · In-and-outs (15)

Training Notes

· Rest minimally between movements to maintain intensity.

· Focus on form, breathing, and muscle engagement over speed.

· Adjust volume as needed to match your current fitness level.

· Consistency and discipline matter more than perfection.

Optional Coaching Tip

Master your body before you try to master weight.

KEEP IT SIMPLE: DO WHAT WORKS FOR YOU

Some trainers are strongly against counting calories and watching the scale. However, you need to focus on what works for you and your individual psyche because my normal and their normal might be abnormal to you. I believe strongly in counting calories because I believe strongly in mathematics; yet, I agree with their notion of scale watching, even though I contradict that philosophy by stepping on the scale frequently throughout the day. We all live in contradictions, so you need to focus on you and what works, rather than following everything I write or others write or say to a science. We are finite human beings, with limited knowledge.

Remember, I am sharing what worked for me, and what I surmise will work for you. I write from a loving and motivating perspective. Your job is to become inspired and take these words and put them into action. You are not obligated to follow any plan or other person's ideas; you are obligated to take control of your life and start living. You must grasp the fact that you do not have time to waste, and you must understand that healthy living can be fun. I believe in you, but it will NOT work if you do not believe in yourself. In order to keep it simple, you must have realistic food goals and work out goals that match your set weight loss or fitness goals. For example, you cannot have a target goal of losing five pounds in two weeks, if you workout twice a week and consume 3,000 calories or more per day.

You could lose five pounds or more if you decided to workout (e.g., intense cardio and weight training) four to five days a week and consuming no more than 1400 calories per day. This is what I mean by simple mathematics; and it would be ideal to eat good fats (i.e., almonds) and clean carbohydrates (i.e., oranges) rather than bad fats (i.e., butter) and bad carbohydrates (i.e., donuts and cakes). When your goals are to procure a hard and lean body, you must be committed to clean eating...it is the only way. Do not be persuaded by this pill and workout video gimmicks. I worked out for years with no significant results. A toned core and bodybuilding abs are developed from a simple diet.

You can buy portion-control containers to preset your amounts prior to a meal. Preparation and organization will help you remain intact and on track to a healthy lifestyle and guaranteed results. I will not lie to you; it requires some commitment and hard work, but it is very doable. I did it, and I am no better than you. I was willing to accept a force greater than myself and believe this lifestyle was possible. The beauty of accepting this philosophy is that this journey becomes a perpetual way of viewing life, so you will not have to worry about the fat coming back. This way of life challenges you to pledge to yourself. Since my significant body transformation, I have indulged way too much in cereal, cakes, donuts, brownies, and other delicacies; but my weight has hovered around 172 because my metabolism is higher now. I also stay devoted to fitness, and more importantly, my body has changed. This change causes me to reject this food, and a cloying experience emerges.

My body is not the same, and in order for me to develop significant fat again, I would require an entrusted effort. Simply put, it would demand work and a conscious effort. Why would I ever do that? My question to you, is why not change your life and follow this path? Ripped abs, a healthy existence, and happiness are hidden inside you, so make a pledge and join the fit body club. I will always be a fat boy in/at heart, and I will always enjoy new foods and desserts when I desire; but I will continuously pull up my shirt to show my abs and walk around shirtless at pools and beaches to exhibit my bodybuilding abs. Enjoy the best of both worlds, all it requires is a lot of sacrifice up front...follow my movement and share this book with your friends.

My Typical Vegetarian Day

Time	Meal / Activity
6:00 AM	Half bottle of water (500 ml) and five-minute meditation
7:00 AM	Cutie (orange), apple, or banana; finish remaining water (500 ml / 17 oz)
9:30 AM	Post-workout: Protein shake (Syntha-6 – vanilla flavor); drink another 500 ml of water
11:00 AM	Snack on almonds (read label; limit to 150 calories or stay within 1500–1700 daily calories); drink another 500 ml of water
1:30 PM	Granola bar (chocolate chip); drink another 500 ml (17 oz) of water

Time	Meal / Activity
4:00 PM	Hummus and carrots or organic chips (limit to 150 calories); drink another 500 ml of water
7:00 PM	Veggie burger, pizza, or similar vegetarian option; drink 500 ml of water
9:00 PM	Green tea and water before bed; if hungry, eat half a palm of almonds

My Typical Non-Vegetarian Day

Time	Meal / Activity
6:00 AM	Half bottle of water (500 ml) and five-minute meditation
7:00 AM	Cutie (orange), apple, or banana; finish remaining water (500 ml / 17 oz)
9:30 AM	Post-workout: Protein shake (Syntha-6) or egg and turkey sausage burrito; drink another 500 ml of water
11:00 AM	Snack on almonds or cashews (limit to 150 calories); drink another 500 ml of water
1:30 PM	Hummus and organic chips (monitor calories); drink another 500 ml of water
4:00 PM	Broccoli and peanut butter (limit to 150 calories); drink another 500 ml of water
7:00 PM	Grilled chicken breast, brown rice, and greens; drink 500 ml of water
9:00 PM	Green tea and water before bed; if hungry, eat half a palm of almonds

My Typical Day After Weight Loss

My relationship with food has changed. I enjoy food, but I no longer overeat. Balance and awareness guide my choices.

Time	Meal / Activity
6:00 AM	Half bottle of water (500 ml) and five-minute meditation
7:00 AM	Cinnamon spice oatmeal; finish bottle of water (500 ml / 17 oz)
9:30 AM	Post-workout: Protein drink or egg and turkey sausage sandwich/burrito; drink another 500 ml of water
11:00 AM	Snack on almonds or fruit; drink another 500 ml of water
1:30 PM	Granola bar (chocolate chip); drink another 500 ml of water
4:00 PM	Two peanut butter and jelly sandwiches; drink another 500 ml of water
7:00 PM	No strict restrictions; practice portion control
9:00 PM	Green tea and water before bed; if hungry, eat half a palm of almonds

Supplement Note
- Daily multivitamin
- B-complex vitamins
- Fish oil

HOW I LOST 13 POUNDS IN 7 DAYS

(I do not recommend this for everyone; it is considered unhealthy and dangerous by some medical professionals)

As you read the heading, I hope you realize that this daunting trek was a spiritual one. This was by far one of the hardest challenges of my existence, but my friends and social media followers kept me inspired throughout the process. First and foremost, it would have been impossible without my unshakeable faith and oneness with God. Some of you might be stuck on my foundation or my source, my oneness with God. Prompting me to define my understanding or belief in God. God is greater than man's constraints (religion) and ideals (finite and human), but at the same time, God can be found in all of those elements.

God is the alpha and omega, and God is the inventor of my spirit, which directs my physical being or flesh. I believe God specifically chose my spirit to exist in my body, and I work incessantly to align my spirit back with God's omnipresence. Some people view God as science or alpha and omega of many religions; and I surmise that many people are referring to the same God but believe in different ways to connect with God's spirit. Personally, I acknowledge Jesus (name as we know it in the U.S.) as the son of the most high, sacrificing his life for the sins of the world. However, I believe that we have the same spirit dwelling in us as Jesus. Why am I sharing my beliefs with you?

This is not to promote religion; I am not a huge fan of organized religion because Jesus was radical and followed God, not traditions and customs of modern religion of his times. Also, God is too grand to be confined and explained in any religion. I embedded this information here to allow you to be privy to my thinking and what led me during my 13 pound challenge. My mind was focused on how to accomplish this lofty task and give God the glory. I had to listen to my spirit to guide me through this process. God sends omens as people, things, numbers, visions, thoughts, etc.; it is our job to listen and allow those divine nuances lead us.

The first nuance was to set **accountability** for myself. This led me to announce my journey on social media, take a picture of the scale and share with others, and tell other people about my formidable task. Some people thought I was crazy and expressed their unbelief in my spoken goal. I learned that our goals must be **spoken** and contrived in a **courageous** fashion that it appears crazy to others; this activates the spiritual realm and calls unseen powers into action. The taxing part of this procedure is to **believe** your spoken goal. Leading your physical temple into action and pushing your body beyond its normal limits.

I meditated, read scripture and a page of a self-help book, and prayed constantly to usher my body during this weight loss venture. Most of this would occur prior to engaging in my morning workouts to set my mind on the right course. Notice that this is a detailed step-by-step method: mind, spirit, and body. It is germane to balance all three components to create oneness with your godly spirit. Once those segments are balanced, you must constantly remind yourself that my body is yours and I will honor you with it.

Now, you must **ask** your godly spirit to discern between the appropriate workouts for your unique body. I was led to workout differently than some of the workouts stated early in this book. I was guided to perform cardio for 25-30 minutes prior to weight training on an empty stomach (no food). I was directed to drink water and recognize the beauty and power within every sip, thanking God as I consumed every drop. This assisted me to maintain a God-conscious and focus during my workouts and seven-day odyssey. Remember, it is not really about you; it is about honoring God and shining brightly to inspire others to be drawn to your godliness, which might lead others to your heavenly father. Back to my workout, after completing cardio, I performed a gauntlet of strength training and core exercises. For example, I worked my biceps and shoulders on Monday.

I morphed into a **busy bee**; a principle I introduced early in this book. I chose a light dumbbell that allowed me to perform 12 reps of standing bicep curls. Employing this exercise with no rests or breaks, I executed 25 reps of in and outs to engage my core muscles. Then, I performed the same workouts again three times before transitioning to a new workout. Shoulders were the next exercise to target in my training; I executed standing shoulder press for 12 reps and immediately, 60-second planks (three additional sets). When I transitioned from these set of exercises, I performed hammer curls in conjunction with shoulder raises (in and outs) with no breaks. In between the workouts, I executed 30 jumping jacks to keep my heart rate elevated and to maintain my fat-burning zone.

I call this total body engagement, giving my body an opportunity to build muscle and cut fat simultaneously. Side-arm hammer curl was the next bicep exercise, and it was performed with a slow squeeze to insinuate the muscle pump (the ball of part of the bicep); inside stadium stairs were done immediately after each set, to maintain my burn and body fat cut. Once again, four sets were executed with each exercise. Thirty minutes of stair climbers followed this workout or thirty minutes of the arc trainer at the completion of my workouts for any given day during this intense seven days. The very last segment of every day was 30-45 minutes of the sauna or steamer to conclude gym sessions. Yet, the hardest part was once I left the gym and decided what to ingest and digest. The **cardinal** part of my workouts is to keep moving and working when your feet make contact with the gym floor.

CHAPTER

13

FOOD IS THY MEDICINE

We are what you consume, and you are shaped by how much you consume; this is the mantra that guided me through this formidable challenge. It would be a lovely world if I could eat as many donuts and cakes as I desired and still had the ability to drop weight and tone up. This is the point when I tell you that that dream does not exist, and it will never exist. However, you can indulge a little, for a day or two and possibly maintain your sculpted physique; this should not become a habitual habit because negative consequences will follow, such as poor decision-making and eating routines will emerge. During this seven-days period, my morning consisted of a bottle of water prior to entering the gym.

When I finished my grueling workout, I consumed two scoops of protein power (22grams of protein per scoop) mixed in eight ounces of water; this became my first tangible meal. I casually drank my protein shake (Syntha-6 Vanilla flavor) on my way to work. Two hours later, I snacked on a hand full of almonds and 20-ounce bottle of water. My third eating time would count as my second meal, and I would tailor it two hours after my first snack. This second meal was extremely simplistic and free of bread and bad sugars; it was approximately five bite sizes pieces of chicken and two tablespoons of carrots concomitant with my obsession of water.

Two hours later, I was eating again. I devoured vegetables, and green beans became my preference. I would ingest green beans until my craving for food subsided. I listened to my mental or God-conscious to inform me when I should continue or discontinue eating any food to tap into my inner God-conscious was crucial for my plight to lose 13 pounds. Another bottle of water accompanied my snack of green beans. My last meal was a peanut butter and jelly sandwich to placate my desire for sugar and bread; I listened to my body and kept my consumption to a minimal. Five out of my seven days consisted of this proverbial ingestion of food; but you must note, that two days were spent on fasting, praying, and meditating, with the consistent workout regime. Another caveat is that I drank hot tea every night prior to bedtime, and I procured at least five to six hours of sleep every night.

Eating patterns remained rote to ensure consistency and reliability on my behalf. I was too afraid to digress and explore new food options. I viewed food as a means to an end, seeing as my medicine to live and to actively engage in life. I never sought to live for food, but I did deviate from my scheduled eating twice; one day my body craved Blaze pizza and a cupcake. I gave into those desires because I do not believe in depriving my body. Deprivation has caused my body to reject my clean eating many times, conjuring up some insidious thoughts that led to the mass consumption of forbidden delicacies. My repudiation of sweets transmute into an ingestion of five personalized red velvet cakes. Allowing myself to partake in those distractions propelled me to add additional workouts to my day; so three days out of the seven days, I worked out twice. Do not worry about working out twice in a day though; you should authorize your body to lead you rather than concentrating on leading your body.

Realize that when you permit your body to guide you, it is godly; but when you attempt to control your body, it is flesh-driven, the antithesis of godliness. I will commence this specialized section with this statement:

Mind, body, and spirit should be the key to acquiring an amazing body or abs like a body builder, and it must become a lifestyle. The pursuit of godliness contrives a lifestyle; the pursuit of vanity creates evilness. One sustains a lifetime, while the later concludes when the ego that drives it dies out.

NGA RIVER CITY CLASSIC 2024

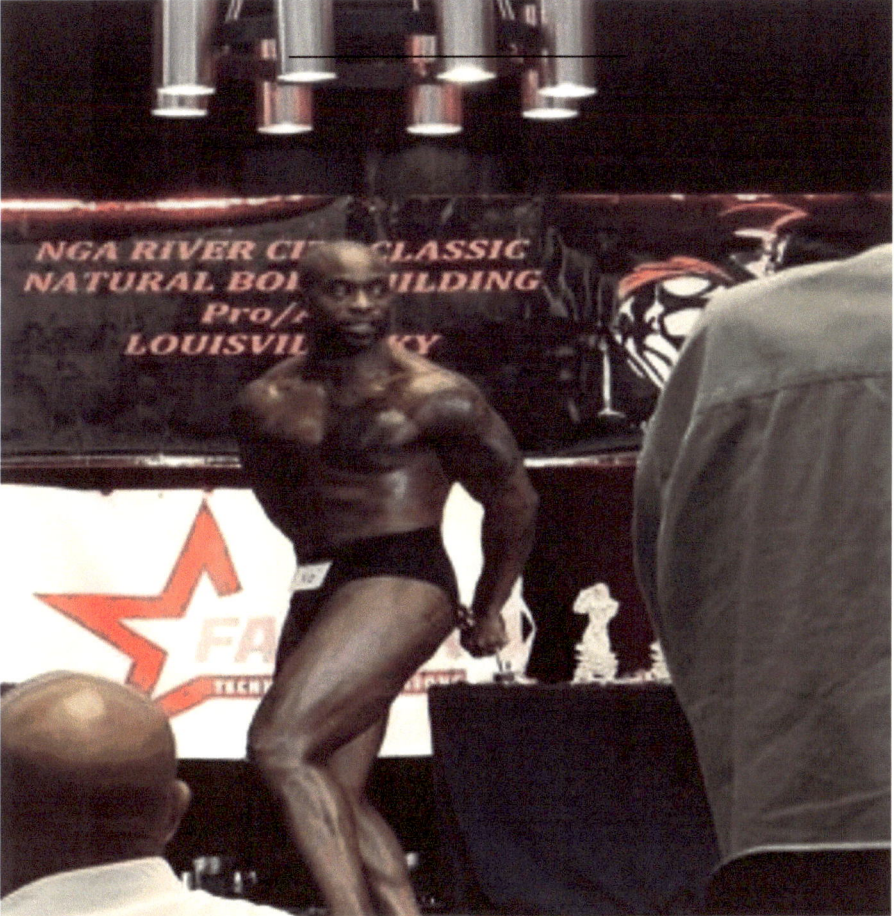

CHAPTER

14

MY ROAD TO OCB PRO

B odybuilding was never on my radar. I respected the discipline, the sacrifice, and the sculpted bodies that came from years of dedication, but it was never something I saw myself pursuing. I enjoyed food, embraced indulgence at times, and lived comfortably within that space. However, my health journey awakened a question I first encountered in graduate school: *What if?* What if I pushed my body harder? What if I delayed gratification? What if I committed to consistent cardio? What if I learned the science behind macros and the art of bodybuilding? Then the pain began. A constant ache in my left hip followed me everywhere—standing, sleeping, running, and playing sports.

Eventually, I learned I needed a total hip replacement. On March 4, 2020, just one week before the world shut down due to COVID, I underwent surgery. That moment changed everything. What followed was a season of deep sadness. The leg that had carried me through college athletics and professional arena football was gone. I felt disconnected from my identity. I knew I had to accept this new reality, but I didn't know how to find peace within it. In silence and prayer, I heard a faint voice say, "You will enjoy the last chapter of your life more than the first." I didn't fully understand it, but I began to believe it. In the summer of 2022, I trained with two individuals, Guill and Will, who introduced me to the true art of bodybuilding. I learned about time under tension, progressive overload, proper hydration, and intentional nutrition. That experience opened my eyes to the difference between casually lifting weights and deliberately building a body.

Something awakened in me. I became curious. Hungry. Focused. I started studying physiques, asking questions, and observing symmetry. I wanted balance. I wanted mastery. One day in that summer of 2023, I asked a former bodybuilder, James Ward, about his biceps. That simple question led him to encourage me to compete in the NGA River City Classic the following year. I laughed and said, "Maybe." But what I really meant was no. A year later, James reached out again and told me he believed I could win. Reluctantly, I agreed to compete, not to win, but to face my fear and add another challenge to my Be Limitless journey. I felt unprepared. I doubted my conditioning and my posing. Still, I stepped on stage, and I won the River City Classic 40+ and open Natural Bodybuilding divisions on June 24th 2024.

Yet I wasn't satisfied. That win ignited something deeper. I sought guidance from local legends like Beano Wallace and Jason Akers. I competed again and again, hearing people tell me I was too old, that winning a pro card so quickly was impossible. Their doubt fueled me. I created a personal challenge called Road to Pro and declared that I would earn my pro card in my hometown of Knoxville, Tennessee. On September 13, 2025, I competed at the OCB Tennessee Natural. It was my seventh show. My competitor number was 13.

That day, I competed in both the 40+ Classic Physique and the Open Classic Physique divisions. I felt confident. I kept hearing a quiet voice say, *You will win.* I told the other competitors, "What God has for you is for you, and no one can take it." This was also my first show under my new legal name, Limitless Williams. When the results were announced for the 40+ division, my name was not called for first place. I was stunned. My confidence collapsed. Backstage, I sat in a chair, pulled my shirt over my head, and questioned everything. Then someone tapped my shoulder and said, "Limitless, remember what you said. What God has for you is for you. You still have the open division." I didn't feel inspired. I felt defeated. But something inside whispered, *Give your best and let God do the rest.* I walked back on stage. The crowd roared. The judges deliberated. When they announced the winner of the Open Classic Physique, they called my name. Competitor number 13. Limitless Williams. I dropped to my knees and whispered, "Thank you." In that moment, I heard God say, *Never doubt Me. You thought it would come the easy way, but I made a way where there was no way.* That day, I learned to never doubt myself, never shrink my dreams, and never underestimate what faith, discipline, and belief can produce.

Think big.
Believe boldly.
Move with faith.
You are Limitless.

CHAPTER 15

7-DAY LEAN MASS & FAT LOSS PLAN GOAL

7- DAY LEAN MASS & FAT LOSS PLAN
Goal: Preserve muscle, strip fat, maintain energy

Calories: ~1,800–2,100/day (adjust based on size/activity)

Protein target: ~1–1.2g per lb of lean body mass

Carbs: Timed around workouts

Fats: Controlled, clean sources

DAILY STRUCTURE (BASELINE)

Meal 1 – Morning

Protein + light carbs

Meal 2 – Mid-Morning

Lean protein + greens

Meal 3 – Post-Workout

Higher carbs + protein

Meal 4 – Afternoon

Protein + vegetables

Meal 5 – Evening

Protein + greens (low carb)

7-DAY MEAL PLAN

DAY 1 – FOUNDATION DAY
Meal 1

- 6 oz ground turkey
- Spinach (sautéed or raw)

Meal 2

- 6 oz chicken breast
- Green beans

Meal 3 (Post-Workout)

- 6 oz salmon
- 1 medium sweet potato

Meal 4

- 6 oz lean ground beef (90/10)
- Spinach

Meal 5

- 6 oz tilapia
- Steamed green beans

DAY 2 – HIGH PROTEIN, LOWER CARB
Meal 1

- 6 oz chicken
- Spinach

Meal 2

· 6 oz ground turkey
· Green beans

Meal 3 (Post-Workout)

· 6 oz steak (sirloin)
· Small sweet potato

Meal 4

· 6 oz tilapia
· Spinach

Meal 5

· 6 oz salmon
· Green beans

DAY 3 – REFEED (Controlled Carbs)
Meal 1

· 6 oz ground turkey
· Sweet potato

Meal 2

· 6 oz chicken
· Spinach

Meal 3 (Post-Workout)

· 8 oz steak
· Sweet potato

Meal 4

- 6 oz salmon
- Green beans

Meal 5

- 6 oz tilapia
- Spinach

DAY 4 – FAT BURN FOCUS
Meal 1

- 6 oz chicken
- Spinach

Meal 2

- 6 oz ground beef
- Green beans

Meal 3 (Post-Workout)

- 6 oz tilapia
- Small sweet potato

Meal 4

- 6 oz salmon
- Spinach

Meal 5

- 6 oz turkey

· Green beans

DAY 5 – POWER DAY
Meal 1

· 6 oz steak
· Spinach

Meal 2

· 6 oz chicken
· Green beans

Meal 3 (Post-Workout)

· 8 oz salmon
· Sweet potato

Meal 4

· 6 oz turkey
· Spinach

Meal 5

· 6 oz tilapia
· Green beans

DAY 6 – CUT & CONDITION
Meal 1

· 6 oz chicken
· Spinach

Meal 2

- 6 oz ground beef
- Green beans

Meal 3 (Post-Workout)

- 6 oz tilapia
- Sweet potato

Meal 4

- 6 oz salmon
- Spinach

Meal 5

- 6 oz turkey
- Green beans

DAY 7 – ACTIVE RECOVERY / RESET
Meal 1

- 6 oz turkey
- Spinach

Meal 2

- 6 oz chicken
- Green beans

Meal 3

- 6 oz steak
- Sweet potato

Meal 4

- 6 oz salmon
- Spinach

Meal 5

- 6 oz tilapia
- Green beans

HYDRATION

- **1–1.5 gallons of water per day**
- Add electrolytes if training hard
- Green tea or black coffee OK

IMPORTANT NOTES

- Season with **herbs, lemon, vinegar, garlic, pepper**
- Avoid sauces, sugar, fried foods
- No alcohol
- Sleep 7–9 hours
- Lift heavy 4–6x/week + light cardio

EXPECTED RESULTS (4–8 weeks)

- Significant fat loss
- Muscle preservation or growth
- Increased vascularity
- Sharpened mental focus

ADVANCED 7-DAY
BODYBUILDING PROGRAM

Goal: Lean mass development, muscle density, conditioning
Training Level: Advanced
Split Type: Push / Pull / Legs + Conditioning
Rest Between Sets: 45–75 seconds
Tempo: Controlled (3–1–1 where possible)

DAY 1 – CHEST & TRICEPS (POWER + PUMP)

Exercise	Sets	Reps	Notes
Barbell Bench Press	4	6–8	Heavy compound
Incline Dumbbell Press	4	8–10	Deep stretch
Cable Fly (mid-level)	3	12–15	Peak contraction

Exercise	Sets	Reps	Notes
Weighted Dips	3	10–12	Lean forward
Rope Pushdowns	3	12–15	Full extension
Overhead DB Extensions	3	12–15	Stretch triceps

Finisher: Push-up burnout × 2 sets

Cardio: 15 min incline walk or stair climber

DAY 2 – BACK & BICEPS (WIDTH + THICKNESS)

Exercise	Sets	Reps
Deadlifts	4	5–6
Wide-Grip Pull-Ups	4	8–12
Seated Cable Rows	3	10–12
Single-Arm Dumbbell Rows	3	10–12
EZ-Bar Curls	3	10–12
Incline DB Curls	3	12–15
Hammer Curls	2	15

Finisher: Battle ropes or rower – 10 minutes

DAY 3 – LEGS (QUADS / HAMSTRINGS / GLUTES)

Exercise	Sets	Reps
Barbell Back Squats	5	6–10
Romanian Dead-lifts	4	8–10
Walking Lunges	3	12 ea.
Leg Press	3	15
Leg Extensions	3	15
Seated Hamstring Curls	3	12
Standing Calf Raises	5	15–20

Finisher: Sled pushes or stair sprints

DAY 4 – ACTIVE RECOVERY / CONDITIONING

Choose 1–2:

- Stair climber (30–40 min)
- Boxing or heavy bag work
- Sprints (10 × 100m)
- Sports-based conditioning

Core Circuit (3 rounds):

- Hanging leg raises × 15
- Russian twists × 20
- Plank × 60 sec

DAY 5 – SHOULDERS & ARMS (DETAIL DAY)

Exercise	Sets	Reps
Standing Military Press	4	6–8
Lateral Raises	4	12–15
Rear Delt Flyes	3	15
Upright Rows	3	10–12
Close-Grip Bench Press	3	8–10
Cable Kickbacks	3	15
Preacher Curls	3	10–12
Cable Curls	2	15

DAY 6 – FULL BODY METABOLIC DAY

Circuit x 4–5 rounds:

Exercise	Reps
Kettlebell Swings	20
Push-Ups	20
Jump Squats	20
Pull-Ups	10
Mountain Climbers	40
Plank	60 sec

Rest 60–90 sec between rounds.

DAY 7 – RECOVERY / MOBILITY

- Stretching (30–40 min)
- Foam rolling
- Light walking
- Breathwork & meditation

CARDIO GUIDELINES

- 4–6 days/week
- 20–40 minutes/session
- Mix steady-state + HIIT
- Fasted cardio optional

NUTRITION PRINCIPLES

- Protein: 1–1.2g per lb lean mass
- Carbs timed around training
- Fats moderate, clean
- Water: 1–1.5 gallons daily

MENTALITY

"Discipline beats motivation every time.
You don't rise to the goal — you fall to the standard you train."

OCB THE TENNESSEE
NATURAL 2025

d to Pro: Dr. Limitles
a PRO!

AUTHOR'S BIO

Dr. Limitless Williams is a scholar, speaker, and professional actor dedicated to helping individuals unlock their fullest potential. He serves as an Associate Professor at the University of Tennessee and is the founder of UNMASKYTP, LLC, where he equips leaders to transform challenge into purpose.

An award-winning author and international thought leader, Dr. Limitless has collaborated with global organizations and Fortune 100 companies, delivered over 70 presentations, and published more than 21 scholarly works. His books include *Check Your Life: Be Limitless*, *From Thug to Scholar*, and *From Flab to Abs*.

From overcoming adversity and homelessness to earning multiple degrees, serving in the U.S. Air Force, and becoming a professional natural bodybuilder, Dr. Limitless embodies resilience, discipline, and growth. Through speaking, coaching, and storytelling, he inspires others to unmask their potential and live without limits.

FIRST SHOW 2024

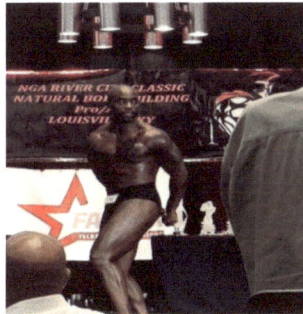

POSING

_____

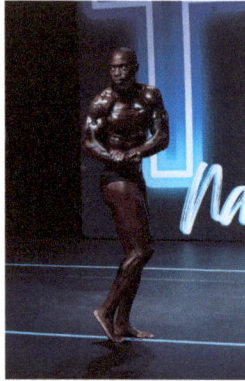

MONSTER MASH 2025

_____

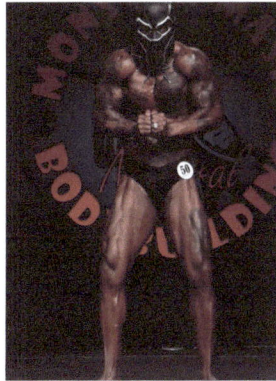

FACE-OFF FOR PRO CARD

_____

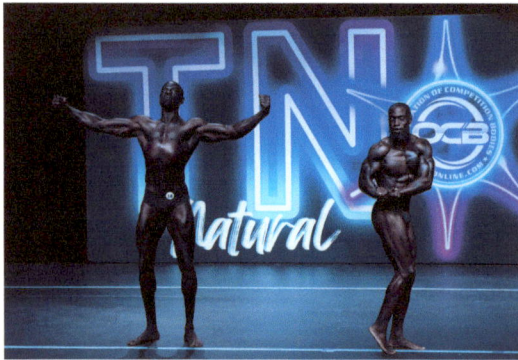

GRATEFUL AND HUMBLED

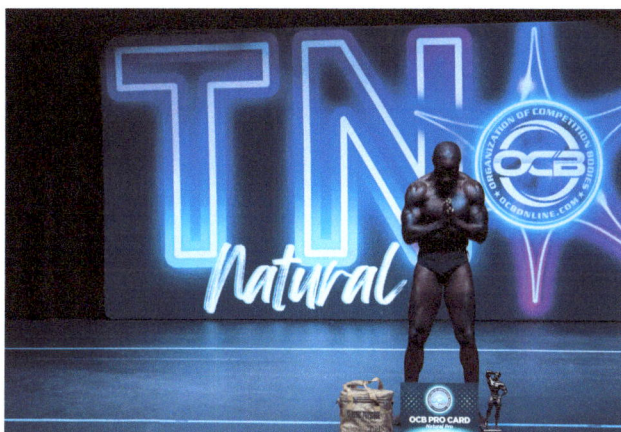

MUSCULAR POSE AT MY
4TH SHOW IN GA

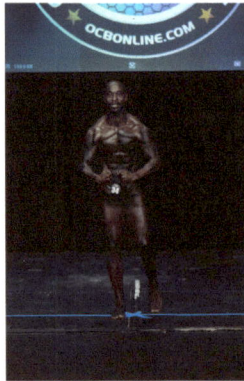

www.ingramcontent.com/pod-product-compliance
Lightning Source LLC
Chambersburg PA
CBHW040933030426
42336CB00006B/66